High Blood Pressure Diet

Diet for Hypertension Free Life!

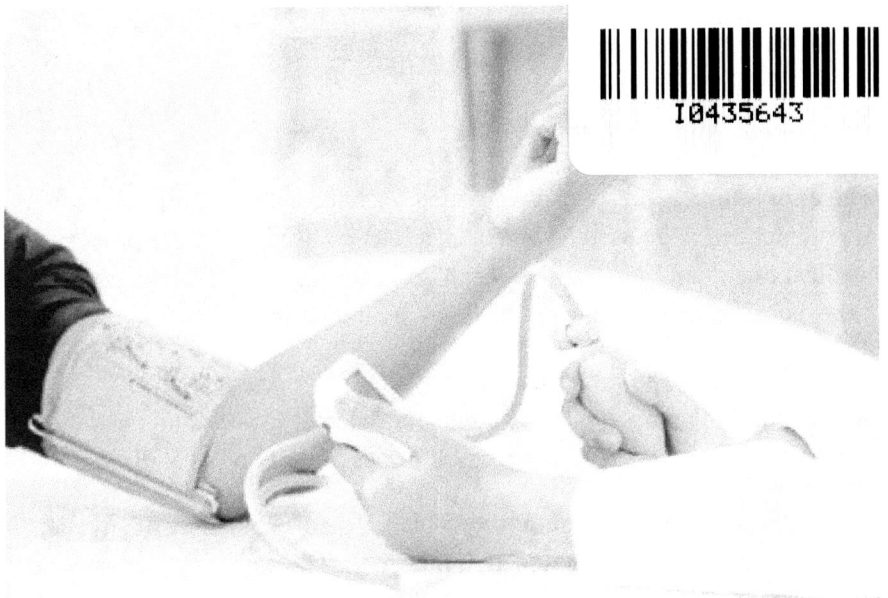

Health Learning Series

M. Usman

Mendon Cottage Books

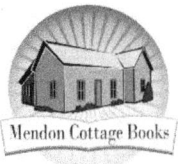

JD-Biz Publishing

Our books are available at

1. Amazon.com
2. Barnes and Noble
3. Itunes
4. Kobo
5. Smashwords
6. Google Play Books

Table of Contents

Prelude

In the United States alone, about 1 in 3 adults suffer from high blood pressure, every year. The condition usually comes without any signs or warnings and a person can be prone to it for years without even knowing about its presence. But, its apparent invisibility does not mean that it sits quietly within one's body; while a person is unaware of it, it wreaks havoc within one's body and damages multiple organs.

Blood pressure, as will be explained in great detail later, is the force that the blood applies on the walls of the arteries as the heart pumps blood in the body. The pressure by which the blood flows can rise or fall, but if it remains high for a long period of time it can start damaging the body. The condition is loosely known as High Blood Pressure.

Knowing your blood pressure numbers is vital, as well as, necessary even if you feel nothing's going wrong. If your blood pressure is normal, no need to worry, but if it is reaching an abnormal level, you may require treatment.

Getting Started

Chapter 1: Overview

Blood pressure is a way of measuring the force exerted by the blood on the walls of the arteries, those that carry blood round the body. The simplest way to analogize the concept behind BP is using a common example. Take a water pump for instance; as the water is pumping though a garden hose, it tries to escape in any direction and to do so it places pressure on the walls. You may increase the pressure on the walls by varying the water control from a faucet or a tap, and in a similar manner the blood pressure on your arteries could buildup if your heart starts pumping at a higher rate. Another way to increase the water pressure is by using thinner pipes; don't worry as no one can sabotage your blood vessels, but they can get clogged which can result in extra material sticking along the arteries, which can once again lead to higher blood pressure.

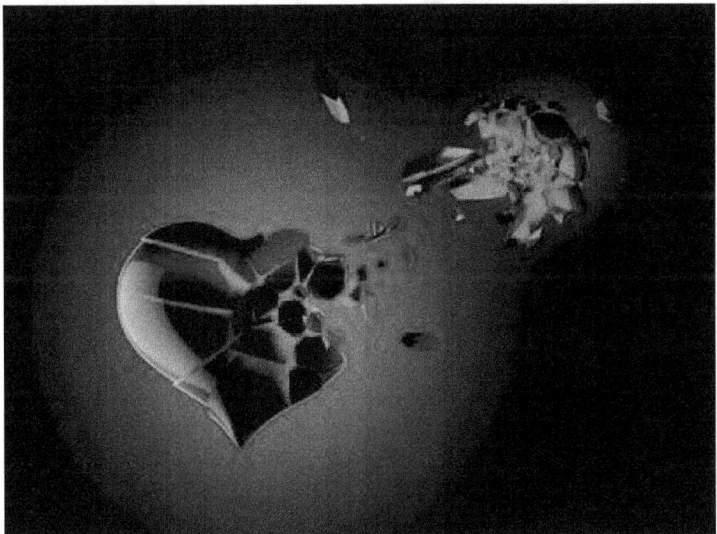

The exact blood pressure is measured with respect to 2 factors.

- Strength of each heartbeat,

- Resistance put up by the vessels through which blood is flowing.

Arterioles are tiny blood vessels that have the greatest control over your blood pressure. They feed into the capillary network, regulating blood pressure, and as they expand/contract in a rhythmic manner, synchronizing with your heart, they become an effective measure to the strength of the muscular tissue of the heart.

The blood pressure is a combination of two different quantities, namely the systolic pressure and the diastolic pressure.

The systolic pressure is measured by taking into account the highest pressure point as the heart contracts and expands. The diastolic pressure is, however, a measurement of the low point of your blood pressure, i.e. when it is at rest. Therefore, medical practitioners pay greater attention to the diastolic pressure as too high values of this pressure mean that the arteries and capillaries are sustaining too much force. This is something they're not designed for when the heart is at rest.

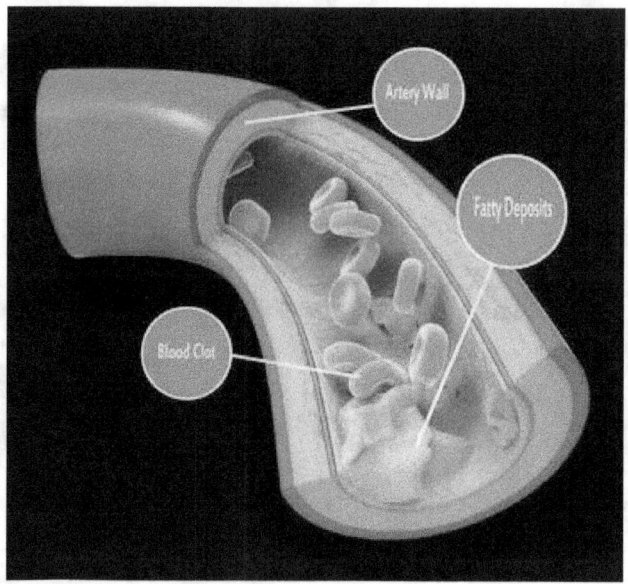

In an average, "non-stressed" adult, the blood pressure would be in the region of 120/80 mmHg; the diastolic pressure continues to fall as you become more athletic or generally less restive throughout your daily activities. Seasoned athletes have a diastolic pressure between 50 and 60. As high blood pressure strikes at a time when most people aren't expecting it, most doctors always check a subject's blood pressure regardless of the ailment he/she complains of.

In technical terminology, high blood pressure is called hyper-tension, but it may be possible that a person suffers from pre-hypertension which has a slight more different definition than the former. According to the US Heart, Lung and Blood Institute:

- A systolic blood pressure between 120 and 139 and a diastolic pressure between 80 and 99 means pre-hypertension.

- A systolic pressure between 140 – 159 along with diastolic pressure between 90 and 99 means stage 1 hypertension.

- A systolic pressure greater than 160 and a diastolic pressure greater than 100 means stage 2 hypertension.

As the book progresses you will learn about the symptoms, causes and prevention techniques of the silent killer that is High Blood Pressure.

Chapter 2: Symptoms

One of the biggest problems that sufferers of this condition face is the lack of clear symptoms associated with the condition. A significant percentage of the populace is left clueless in the face of high blood pressure that only adds to the number of problems that they may soon face.

Still there are a few signs that may help a person judge as to whether he/she suffers from high blood pressure or not. People with elevated levels of blood pressure may experience:

i.   Headaches

ii.   Blurred vision, at times

iii.   Dizziness

iv.   Nausea

v.   Vomiting

vi.   Shortness of breath

vii.   Chest pains

Usually, people let these signs go unnoticed and wakeup only after the body goes through something more major and chronic.

Nominal symptoms of high blood pressure include nosebleeds and it is only logical that high blood pressure would lead to weaker blood vessels which would increase their chances to rupture. Similarly, unexpected dizziness on a frequent basis is another sign of high blood pressure, as a normal person does not experience that. Even if it's not blood pressure, it would be better to report to a doctor rather than self-diagnosing.

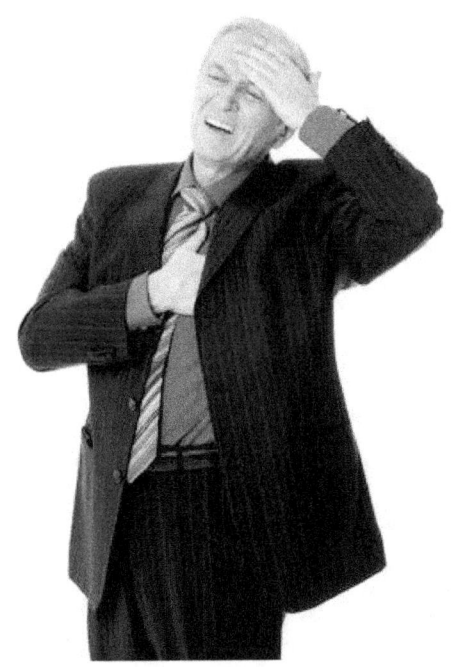

When high blood pressure is left unaddressed for a long period of time, no matter what the reason is, the person can go through problems which certainly result in a trip to the hospital. The long term, chronic signs and effects of high blood pressure include:

i.   Heart attack

ii.   Stroke

iii.   Heart failure

iv.   Kidney failure

v.   Eye damage

Thus, to protect yourself from a series of bigger ailments and conditions, it is advised that you arrange frequent visits to the doctor just to be extra careful.

Chapter 3: Effects of High Blood Pressure

To get a basic overview of the long-term effects of high blood pressure, read the following phrase; "The heart never sleeps".

This phrase alone would be enough to explain to you the importance of the well-being of the whole cardiovascular system. If the heart never sleeps, then that means that the blood vessels connected to the heart (and that mean all blood vessels!) are also active 24/7/365. High blood pressure means that at any instant, any of the countless arteries and veins could burst and flood any major organ with an excess amount of blood.

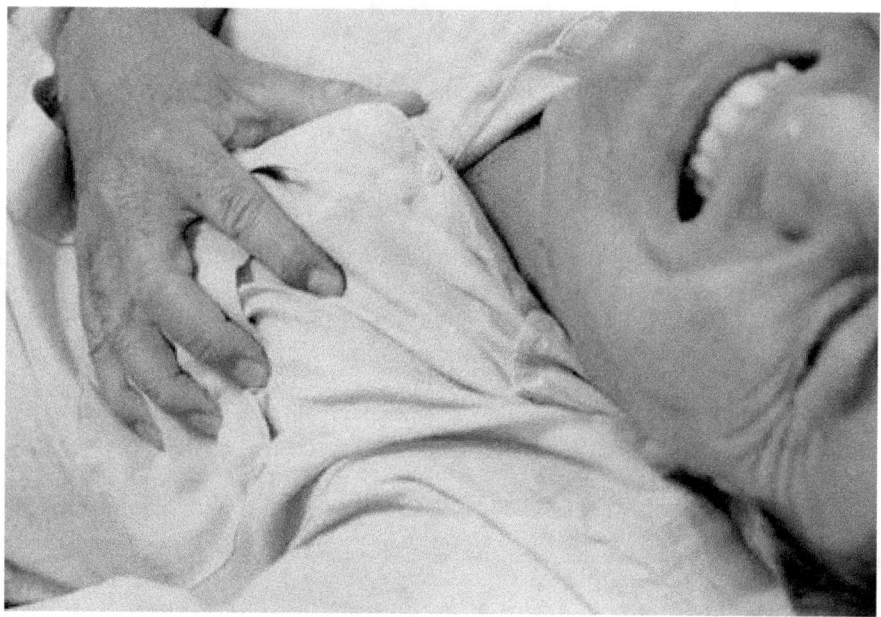

As every single millimeter of the body is covered with a vast network of blood vessels, no part of it is safe when suffering from high blood pressure. The following are a few problems in detail that can be caused due to high blood pressure:

1. **Cardiovascular and/or Heart disease:**

    Heart attacks are the leading cause of death in the United States. Cardiovascular disease claims a single victim every 35 seconds, with 2500 US citizens dying every day due to it. As blood is pumped from the heart, the source of many problems, due to which high blood pressure is caused, lies in one's heart. The most obvious example is a heart attack, in which the heart simply gives up and refuses to pump blood at a higher rate. The fact that the heart has to pump blood at a higher rate means that as time passes it will become stiffer and much thicker, which makes it less capable of doing the job it is originally designed for. This then leads to heart problems including heart attacks and heart failures. Another alternate scenario is that when the heart becomes larger in size, and because of the increased blood pressure, it becomes inefficient at pumping blood. This increases the risk of a heart attack along with a plethora of other problems due to the enlarged size of the heart.

2. Brain Problems:

Brain conditions, like strokes, aren't far behind the common causes of death in the US; they land third. Uncontrolled blood pressure can result in damaged, decreased size of blood vessels in the brain, which in turn, increases the risk of a blood vessel bursting and causing internal bleeding. If a blood vessel gets blocked or bursts, a certain part of your brain won't get the blood it needs to function, and it would either cease functioning temporarily or permanently die. The part of the brain might be a less useful one or the central one, so the risk of you dying as well is in the hands of the strength of the blood vessel.

Blood failure in the brain therefore causes frequent headaches and dizziness, so a trip to the doctor should be number 1 on your to-do-list if you ever experience such conditions. Along with these conditions, you may also suffer from blurred vision, weakness, and inability to talk. Moreover, a person may experience dementia as a result of high blood pressure known as vascular dementia. This condition occurs when a certain part of the brain is damaged from irregular blood flow which leads to loss in memory, loss of speech, and confusion.

3. Kidney Problems:

Kidneys filter your blood of unwanted, toxic and wasteful products and discharge them from your body. If, due to some reason, the kidneys lose their ability to perform at peak efficiency or in worst case, at all, an array of problem may result. Just think for yourself, if the blood is not cleansed of unwanted materials they may flow freely in the body causing additional problems in an already unfavorable environment.

4. Limbs and Eyes:

As no functioning part of the body is free of blood vessels, the damage due to high blood pressure is not limited to internal organs. High blood pressure can also damage the limbs and eyes, which are of great importance, just like other organs.

If your doctor diagnoses you with high blood pressure, they will often investigate the blood vessels located at the back of your eye. The capillaries on the back of your eyes are the only vessels visible so they are immediately investigated for signs of high blood pressure. If they have abnormally expanded and/or exploded, there is a high chance that your eye sight may have been negatively affected.

Coming to the mobility organs, high blood pressure can lead to swollen ankles as well as limbs. This happens when the heart pumps blood at a higher rate, which leads to the accumulation of blood in the ankles, or lower region of the legs. In short term, they may not cause any harm or worry, but in the long run they can lead to much serious problems like varicose veins, venous ulcers and cellulites.

Sufferers of high blood pressure may experience cramping in the legs or ankles which goes away when they are at rest. This could be a result of arterial disease which causes narrowing of the blood vessels located in and around the limbs hence causing pain whenever they come to motion.

5. Other problems:

There are some other particular problems for both men and women that may result from high blood.

Men who suffer from high blood pressure may go through erectile dysfunction as a result of damage to the arteries that transport blood to the genital organs.

Furthermore, as a result of pregnancy, women may suffer from high blood pressure, which may last for several weeks after birth. This type of blood pressure is usually temporary and may not be much of a risk, however if the mother suffered from high blood pressure before getting pregnant, she may have to seek extra medical advice, just to be on the safe side.

Chapter 4: Causes of High Blood Pressure

If high blood pressure persists for a lengthy amount of time it is known as hypertension. Hypertension can then again be divided into 2 more types:

i.   Essential or primary hypertension

ii.   Secondary hypertension

According to the US Heart Association, primary hypertension has no major identifiable cause, but secondary hypertension is much easier to determine.

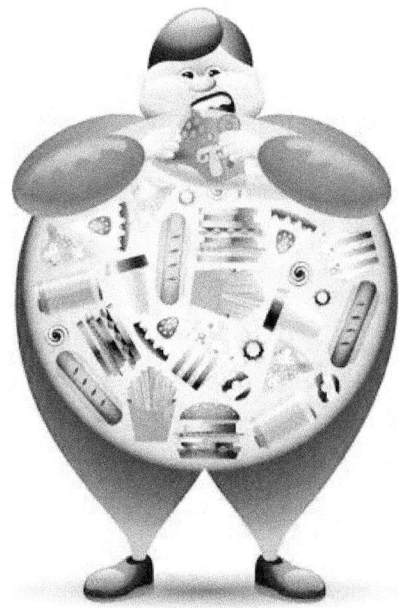

Still doctors are able to identify cases of primary hypertension by hypothesizing the factors that help the onset of the condition. The following are a few factors which are commonly used by medical practitioners:

i.   **Being obese or overweight:**

        Naturally, the more you weigh the more massive you are and the harder it is for the heart to pump blood through your veins. This increases your blood pressure and thus increases the pressure applied by the blood on the arterial walls, as more than the normal amount of oxygen and nutrients are required to keep the obese body working.

ii.   Sleep apnea:

Sleep apneas are the brief instances of time when you are unable to breathe while asleep; it is considered a contributing factor to high blood pressure and is also something susceptible in obese individuals.

iii.   Activity:

As stated in the beginning chapters, the level of activity throughout your daily life can greatly contribute to your level of blood pressure. If you are inactive or do not indulge in exercise, you heart rate will increase and with that, the amount of work needed to pump blood through your arteries.

iv.   Genetics:

If you are mobile, healthy and up to the mark in all walks of life but still have high blood pressure, it can mean only one thing; high blood pressure is present in your genetic structure. It is a fact that high blood pressure can be passed from generation to generation and can show up unexpectedly in a completely normal person.

v.   Tobacco:

Smoking can become a factor in contributing to high blood pressure. Certain chemicals in cigarettes can damage the blood vessels which can increase the blood pressure.

vi.   Alcohol:

Excessive alcohol consumption can weaken the heart, and increase the risk of high blood pressure.

vii.   Mineral consumption:

Too much sodium is not good for the body; excessive intake can increase the amount of fluid retention in the body and thus increase the blood pressure.

On the other hand, very low intake of potassium can elevate the level of sodium in the cells of the body, which can once again lead to high blood pressure.

Next is secondary hypertension, which is caused by pre-existing medical conditions like renal stenosis or heart problems like aortic coarctation. In secondary hypertension it is more than likely that a medical condition causes high blood pressure; this medical condition is then treated which acutely deals with the problem of high blood pressure. It cannot be said that this lessens the severity of high blood pressure, and it can be stated that secondary hypertension can be managed far more easily than primary hypertension.

DASH Diet

While many diets have surfaced that aim to solve the issue of hypertension or high blood pressure, one particular diet that highlights the use of natural products to treat the problem is the "Dietary Approaches to Stop Hypertension Diet". The DASH diet lays particular emphasis on size per meal, types of foods, and their quality, to decrease one's blood pressure. The diet is a lifelong approach to healthy eating designed to keep high blood pressure under check. The diet's fundamental principle is to reduce the amount of sodium in one's diet to counter the effects of high blood pressure. By following the DASH diet, you may be able to bring down your high blood pressure by a few points within a few weeks' time. Over time, your systolic blood pressure will drop, which will drastically increase your quality of life.

Because the DASH diet is a healthy way to eat, its benefits range much wider than just controlling blood pressure. It can improve conditions like osteoporosis, cancer risk, stroke and diabetes.

Sodium Levels:

The DASH diet emphasizes on fruits, vegetables and low fat dairy, along with whole grains, fish and poultry in moderation. There are 2-sodium versions of the diet and it is up to you, as to the one you want.

i.   Standard DASH diet – consumption of 2300 milligrams of sodium per day is allowed.

ii.   Lower Sodium version – consumption of 1500 milligrams of sodium a day is allowed.

Both versions of the diet still allow less sodium than the average amount consumed which is a whopping 3500 mg.

What to eat:

Both versions of the DASH diet include equal amounts of whole grains, veggies, and fruits along with low-fat dairy products. A detailed overview of the types of foods allowed by the diet is as follows:

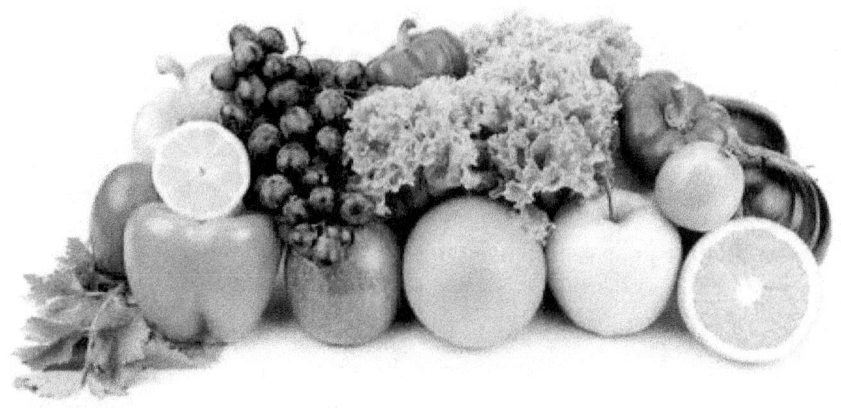

✓ **Grains: 6-8 servings a day.**

Grains like bread, rice, cereal and pasta are allowed by the DASH diet. Examples of a single serving of grain include a slice of whole wheat bread, or a ½ cup cooked rice, pasta, etc.

- Focus on whole grains as they contain more fiber and nutrients compared to the refined grains.

- Grains are naturally low in fat so there is no special need to add butter, cream or cheese to them.

✓ **Vegetables: 4-5 servings a day.**

Tomatoes, broccoli, carrots, greens, sweet potatoes and other vegetables full of fiber, vitamins, and minerals are very good for the heart. Examples of one serving of vegetables include 1 cup raw vegetables or ½ cup cut up vegetables.

- Vegetables aren't side dishes and should be seen as a major component of a meal.

- Fresh or frozen vegetables are both good for your health. When buying canned or frozen vegetables choose those that are labeled "low sodium".

✓ **Fruits: 4-5 servings a day.**

Many fruits need little preparation to become a healthy part of a snack. Like vegetables, they're packed with potassium, magnesium and fiber. A serving of fruit may be 1 medium fruit, ½ cup frozen or canned fruit or 4 ounces of juice.

- Enjoy a piece of fruit with meals, like a snack, and finally round out your day with a dessert made of fresh fruits with a splash of low-fat yogurt.

- Keep the edible peels on the fruit if possible as they are packed with many healthy nutrients.

✓ **Dairy: 2-3 servings a day.**

Milk, cheese, yogurt, etc. are the major sources of calcium, vitamin D and protein in one's diet. The key, however, is to make sure that you choose the dairy products that are low in fat. A sample serving of dairy is 1 cup skimmed milk, 1 ½ oz. cheese or 1 cup yogurt.

- Low fat frozen yogurt can provide a great boost in the total daily intake of dairy products while at the same time offering a sweet treat.

- Choose lactose free products if you experience trouble digesting dairy products.

✓ **Meat, poultry and fish: Less than 7 servings a day.**

Meat is a great source of B-vitamins, iron, zinc and most importantly protein. But even lean varieties contain cholesterol and fat, so it is advisable to cut down the consumption of meat by one third or one half and fill them by vegetables instead. Examples of one serving include 1 oz. skinless poultry, lean meat, etc.

- Trim away any skin and fat from meat and then either roast or grill it instead of frying it in fat.

- Eat fish like tuna, herring, and salmon as they are high in omega-3 fatty acids which help lower cholesterol.

✓ **Nuts, legumes and seeds: 4-5 servings a week.**

Sunflower seeds, kidney beans, almonds, lentils, peas, etc. are all great sources of magnesium, protein, and potassium. They're full of phytochemicals and fiber which are compounds that protect against cancers and other harmful diseases. Serving sizes are usually small like once a day.

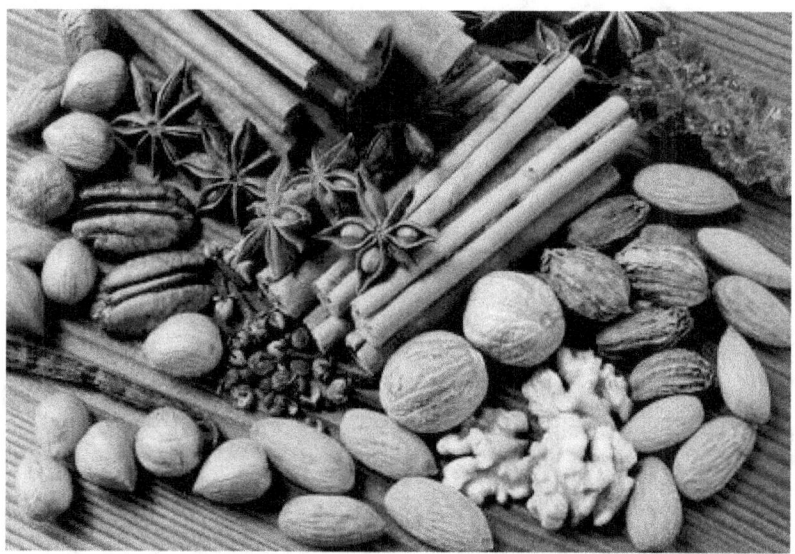

- Nuts sometimes get a bad reputation for their fat content, but it must be known that they contain healthy fats; although they are high in calories, so eat them in moderation.

- Soybean based products like Tempeh and tofu can be great alternatives to meat as they contain all the compounds you get from a serving of meat.

✓ **Fats and oils: 2-3 servings a day.**

Fats help the body absorb essential vitamins and help the immune system work at full notch. But, too much intake of fat leads to an increased risk of obesity, heart disease, and diabetes. One serving of DASH diet includes 1 teaspoon soft margarine, 2 tablespoons salad dressings, and 1 tablespoons mayonnaise.

- Avoid Trans-fats that are found in processed foods.

- Read food labels before purchasing margarine and salad dressing so you can be sure that you are purchasing items with the lowest amount of saturated fat.

✓ **Sweets: Fewer than 5 a week.**

Examples of one serving of sweets include 1 tablespoon of sugar, ½ cup sorbet, and 1 cup lemonade.

- When you eat sweets, make sure you choose non-fat ones.

- Cut back on added sugar as it has no nutritional worth.

Recipes

Chapter 1: Chicken Charred Tomato & Broccoli Salad

Makes: 6 servings

Active time: 40 minutes

Total time: 1 hour

Ingredients:

- 1 ½ pounds skinless, boneless chicken breasts OR 3 cups shredded cooked chicken breast

- 1 ½ pounds medium tomatoes

- 4 cups broccoli florets

- 1 teaspoon salt

- 2 + 3 teaspoons extra-virgin olive oil

- 1 teaspoon freshly ground pepper

- ¼ lemon juice

- ½ teaspoon chili powder

Directions:

Place the chicken in a skillet and add enough water so that it is completely covered. Bring the water to a simmer over high heat. Cover and reduce the heat, allowing it to simmer gently until the chicken is thoroughly cooked and no longer pink; this will take 10 to 12 minutes. Transfer the chicken onto a cutting board, and when cool enough to handle properly, shred using two forks into bite-sized portions. Next, bring a large pot of water to boil and add the broccoli to it, cooking it for 3-5 minutes so that it turns tender; drain and rinse the cold water until it is cool. Meanwhile, take the tomatoes and cut them into halves. Gently squeeze the seeds and discard them; set the tomatoes on paper towels and drain them for 5 minutes. Place a large skillet over high heat and let it heat until it is very hot. Brush the cut sides of the tomatoes with a tablespoon of oil and place them on the pan. Cook until they are charred which will take 4-5 minutes. Brush the tops of the tomatoes lightly with 1 teaspoon oil; turn and cook them until their skin is charred, 1-2 minutes more. Let them cool on a plate but do not clean the pan. Heat the remaining 3 tablespoons oil in the pan over medium-high heat. Add in the pepper, chili powder and salt, cooking while stirring constantly for 45 seconds. Slowly pour in the lemon juice and remove the pan from heat. Coarsely chop the tomatoes and combine them in a single bowl with the shredded chicken that had been prepared earlier; toss to coat. You may cover and refrigerate the dish for up to 2 days.

Chapter 2: Tomato & Olive Stuffed Portobello Caps

Makes: 4 servings

Active time: 35 minutes

Total time: 40 minutes

Ingredients:

- 2/3 cup plum tomatoes, chopped

- ½ cup shredded partly skimmed mozzarella cheese

- 1 teaspoon minced garlic

- ¼ cup chopped Kalamata olives

- 2 teaspoons extra virgin olive oil

- ½ teaspoon chopped rosemary

- 4 Portobello mushroom caps

- 1/8 teaspoon freshly ground pepper

- 2 tablespoons lemon juice

- 2 teaspoons soy sauce

Directions:

Combine the tomatoes, olives, garlic, cheese, rosemary, 1 teaspoon of oil and pepper in a small bowl. Preheat a grill to medium and discard the mushroom stems. Remove the brown grills using a spoon and discard them. Mix the remaining 1 teaspoon of oil, soy sauce and lemon juice in a bowl and brush the mixture over both sides. Oil the grill rack and place the caps on it; cover and grill until they are soft which will take about 5 minutes each side. Remove from the grill and fill it with the mixture prepared earlier.

Return to the grill and cook again until the cheese is melted (3 minutes). Serve.

Chapter 3: Lasagna Rolls

Makes: 6 servings

Active time: 45 minutes

Total time: 45 minutes

Ingredients:

- 1 tablespoon extra-virgin olive oil

- 12 lasagna noodles, preferably whole wheat

- 3 cloves minced garlic

- 1 14 ounce extra-firm water packed tofu

- 3 cups spinach, chopped

- 2 tablespoons finely chopped olives

- ½ cup Parmesan cheese, shredded

- ¼ teaspoon salt

- ¼ teaspoon crushed red pepper

- A 25 ounce jar of marinara sauce

- ½ cup shredded mozzarella cheese

Directions:

Bring a large pot filled with water to boil and cook the lasagna according to the instructions provided on the package. Drain, rinse and put in the pot, covered with cold water. Meanwhile, take a non-stick skillet and heat oil in it over medium heat. Add garlic and stir until fragrant. Next add spinach and tofu and continue to cook along with stirring until the spinach wilts; this will take 3-4 minutes. Transfer the contents of the skillet to a bowl and add in the olives, parmesan, 2/3 cup marinara sauce, salt and red pepper. Wipe out the pan and pour in 1 cup of the marinara sauce.

To make the rolls, place a noodle on the work surface and add ¼ cup of the filling to it. Roll up and place it seam side down in the pan. Repeat the previous steps with the remaining noodles. Spoon some of the marinara sauce over the rolls. Place this pan over high heat and cover it until it simmers. Reduce the heat to medium and let it simmer for 3 minutes. Next, sprinkle the rolls with mozzarella cheese and cook while keeping it covered, until the cheese is melted or for 1 – 2 minutes. Serve while they are still hot. Furthermore, you may store the cooked rolls in a freezer for a month.

Chapter 4: Red Curry

Makes: 4 servings

Active time: 40 minutes

Total time: 40 minutes

Ingredients:

- 4 teaspoons canola oil

- A 14 ounce extra-firm tofu package, rinsed and dried

- 1 pound sweet potatoes, cut into small cubes

- A 14 ounce coconut milk can

- 1-2 teaspoons of red Thai curry paste

- ½ cup vegetable broth

- 1 tablespoon brown sugar

- ½ pound green beans

- ½ teaspoon salt

- 2 teaspoons lime juice

- 1/3 cup chopped fresh cilantro

- 1 lime

Directions:

Heat 2 teaspoons of oil in a large non-stick skillet over medium heat and add tofu to it; cook, stirring every 2 minutes until it is browned. Let it cook for 6 to 8 minutes and then transfer the contents onto a plate. Heat the remaining 2 teaspoons of oil over medium heat and add sweet potato to it. Cook while stirring until the potatoes are browned which will take 4 – 5 minutes. Add coconut milk, curry paste, and broth to taste and bring to a boil. Reduce the heat so it can simmer and cook until the potatoes are just tender. After 4 minutes, add the beans, tofu and brown sugar and cook until the green beans are tender. Add in the salt and the lime juice and sprinkle some cilantro.

Chapter 5: Chicken & Vegetable Curry

Makes: 4 servings

Active time: 35 minutes

Total time: 45 minutes

Ingredients:

- 2 teaspoons canola oil

- 1 medium onion

- 1 medium red bell pepper

- 1 tablespoon minced fresh ginger

- 1 clove garlic

- 1-2 teaspoons red curry paste

- 1 cup reduced-sodium chicken broth

- 1 pound boneless, skinless chicken (breasts)

- 1 cup coconut milk

- 1 tablespoon fish sauce

- 1 ½ cup cauliflower florets

- 1 tablespoon lime juice

- 2 cups baby spinach

- Lime wedges

Directions:

Heat the oil in a large non-stick skillet over medium heat and add onion and bell peppers. Cook with occasional stirs until the contents begin to soften; this will take about 4 minutes. Add ginger, garlic and curry paste and stir. Next, add the chicken and cook while stirring until it is fragrant; this will take about 2 minutes. Stir in the coconut milk, broth, fish sauce and brown sugar, bringing to a simmer. Add the cauliflower and reduce the heat, letting it simmer. Add in the lime juice and spinach and keep cooking until the spinach wilts. Serve along with lime wedges.

Conclusion

By now you must have gained enough knowledge to categorize the dangers of high blood pressure and ways to stop it from completely destroying each part of your body. As every active part of the body requires blood to function, a condition of high blood pressure is bound to affect each corner of the body and can cause serious, life threatening conditions. Millions of people aren't even aware of the disease and leave themselves on its mercy; therefore it is best to keep monitoring your health and visit the doctor regularly to make sure you aren't consumed by the disease before it is too late. The ways, methods, and techniques to protect you from the condition have been given in the book so follow them and lead a better life.

Best of Luck!

References

http://www.fotolia.com/id/47136007

http://www.fotolia.com/id/53256130

http://www.fotolia.com/id/47849169

http://www.fotolia.com/id/48701190

http://www.fotolia.com/id/35435335

http://www.fotolia.com/id/42606253

http://www.fotolia.com/id/45901427

http://www.fotolia.com/id/36637153

Author Bio

Muhammad Usman is a distinguished medical graduate of Allama Iqbal medical college (AIMC). He is a professional writer who has been in the field for more than 4 years. During this time he has produced 10,000+ articles, blogs and eBooks on various niches related to diseases, health, fitness, nutrition and well-being. He is a regular contributor to several journals related to medicine and surgery. He is the editor of several journals and newspapers.

Check out some of the other JD-Biz Publishing books

Gardening Series on Amazon

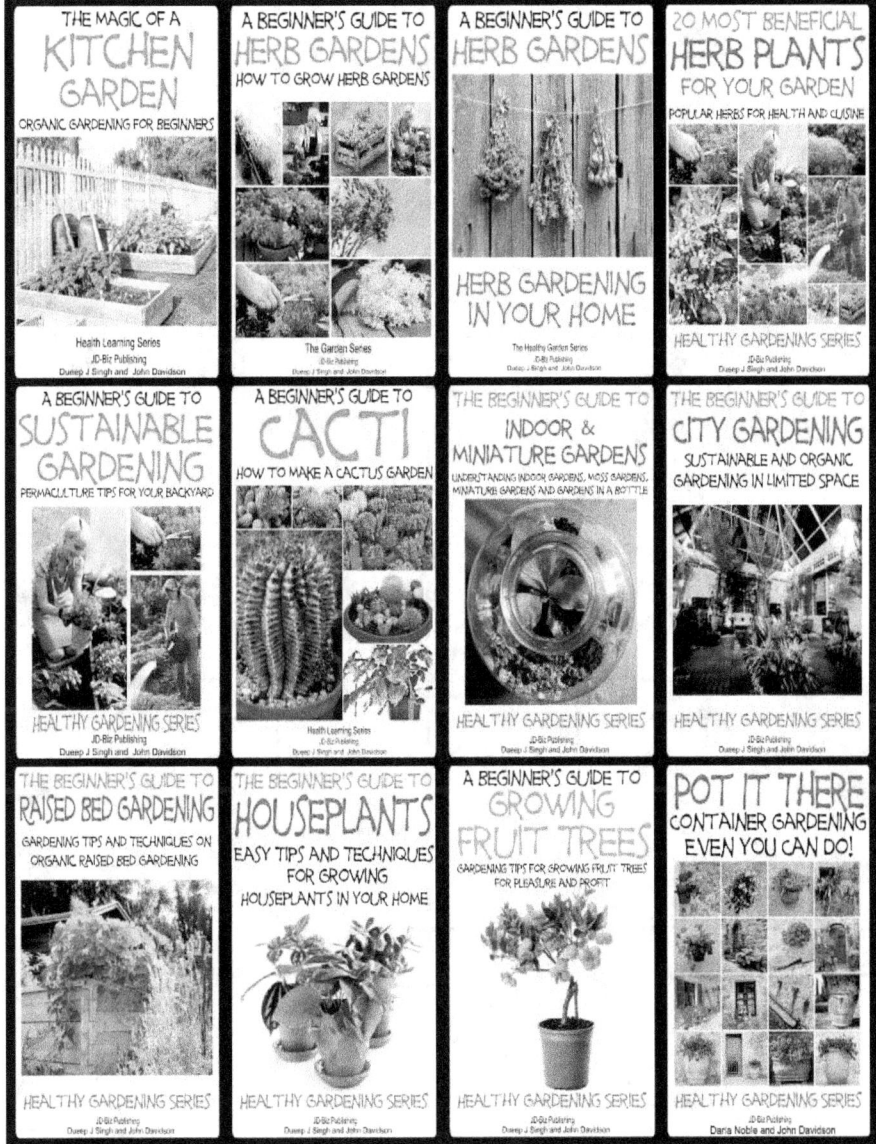

Health Learning Series

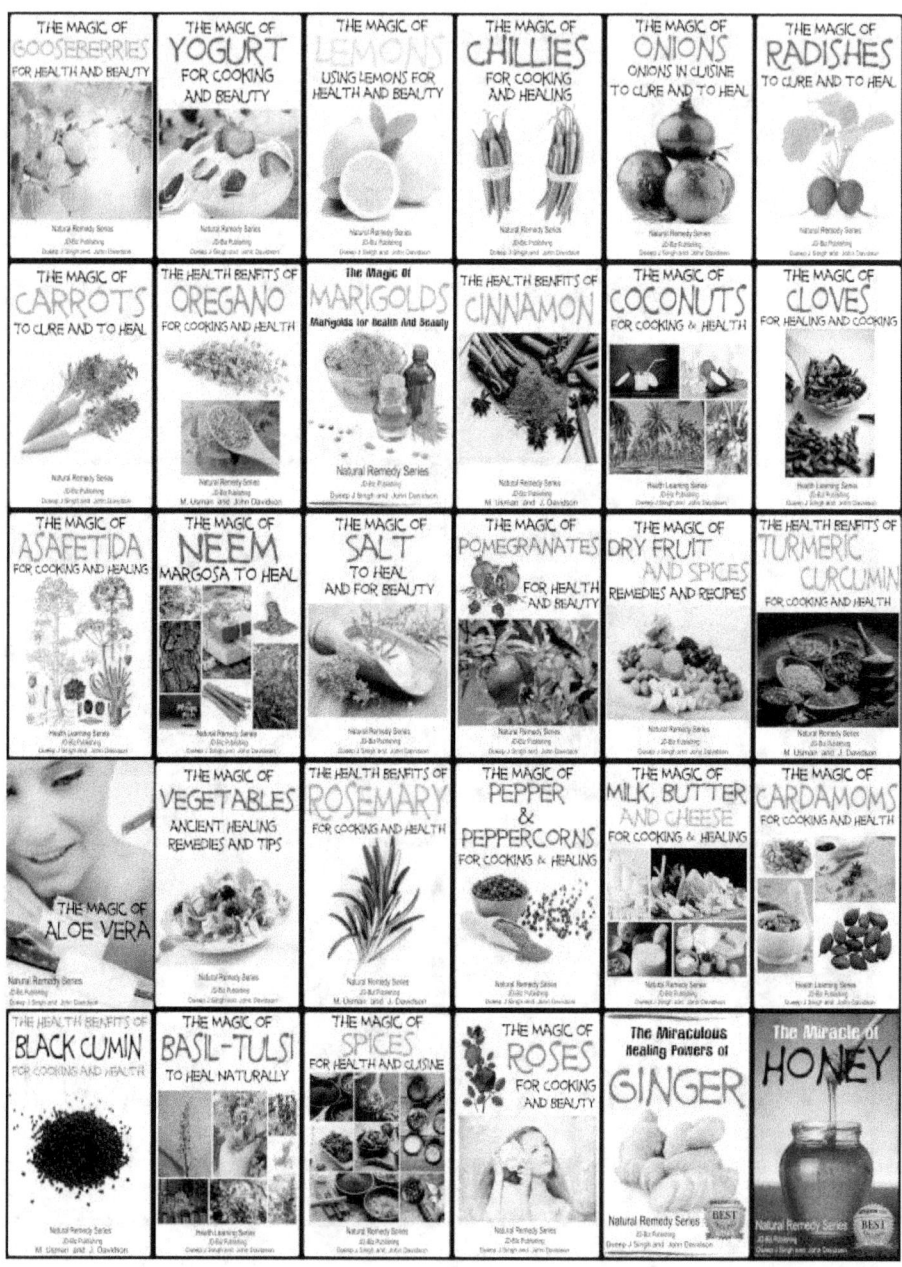

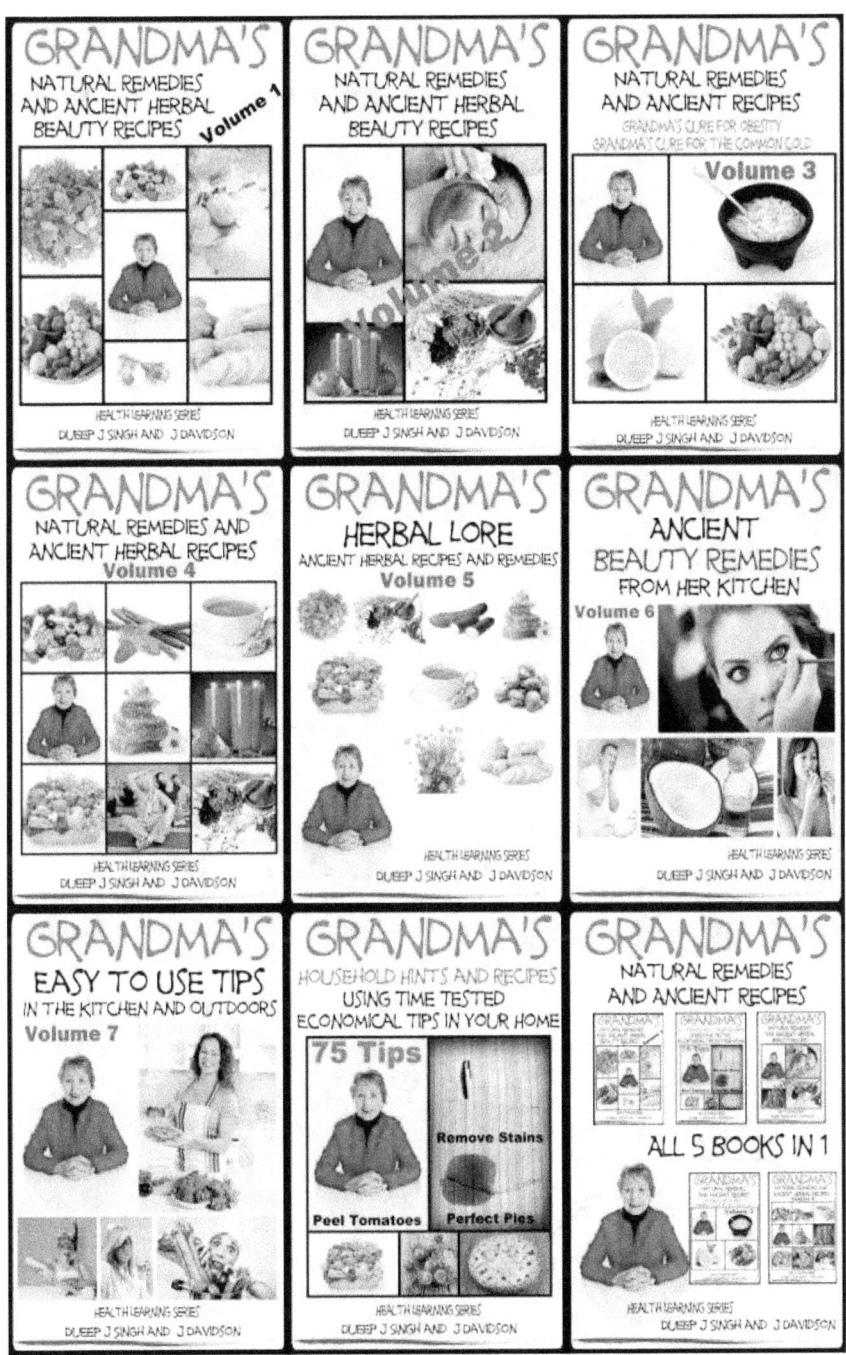

Country Life Books

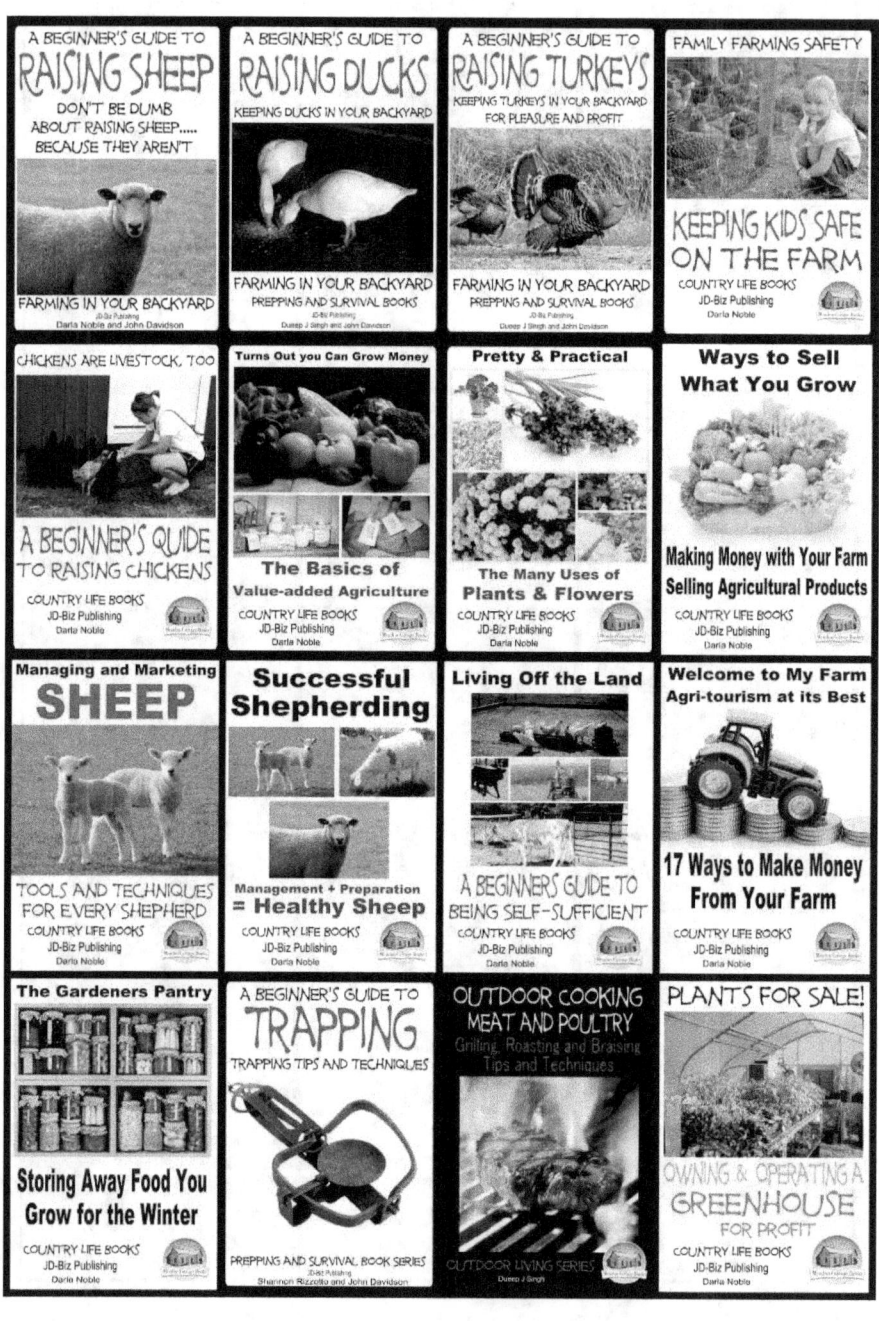

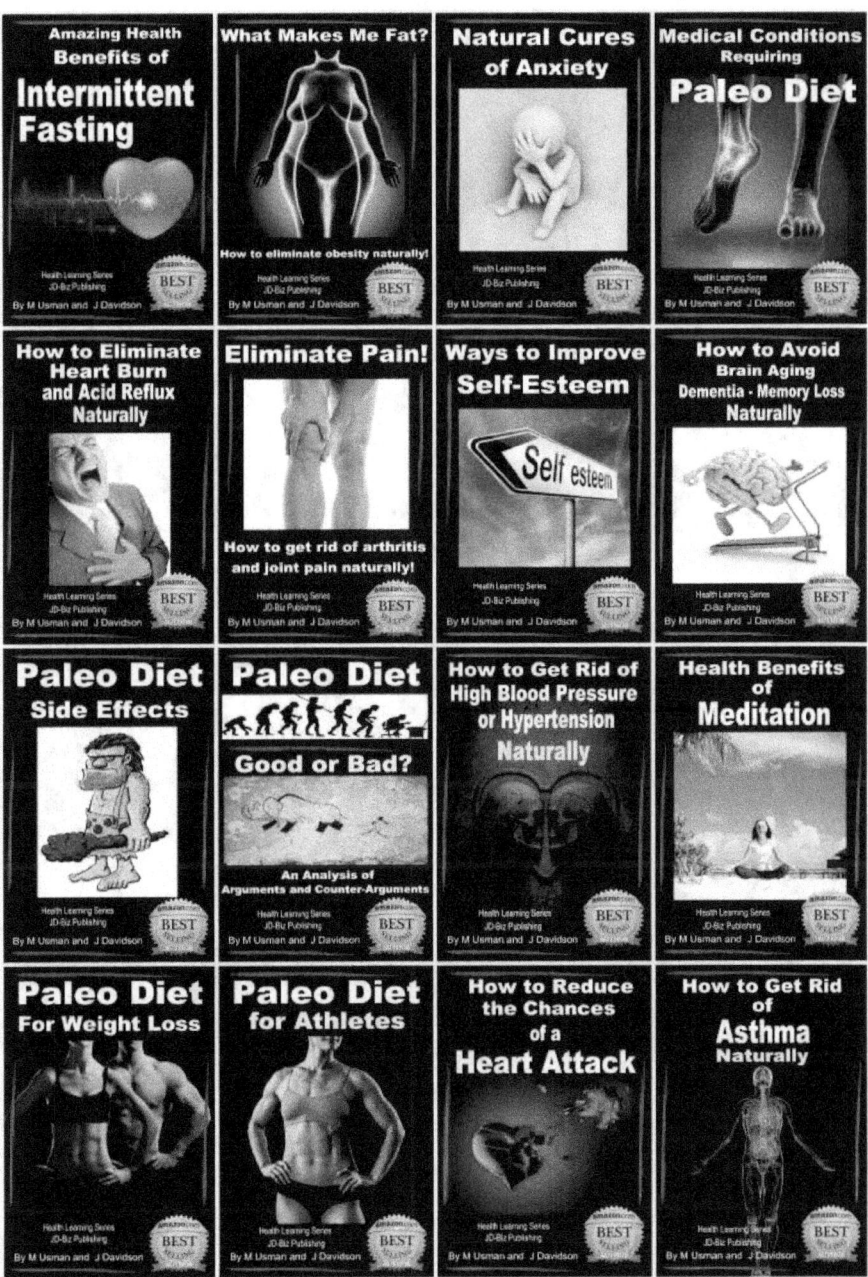

Amazing Animal Book Series

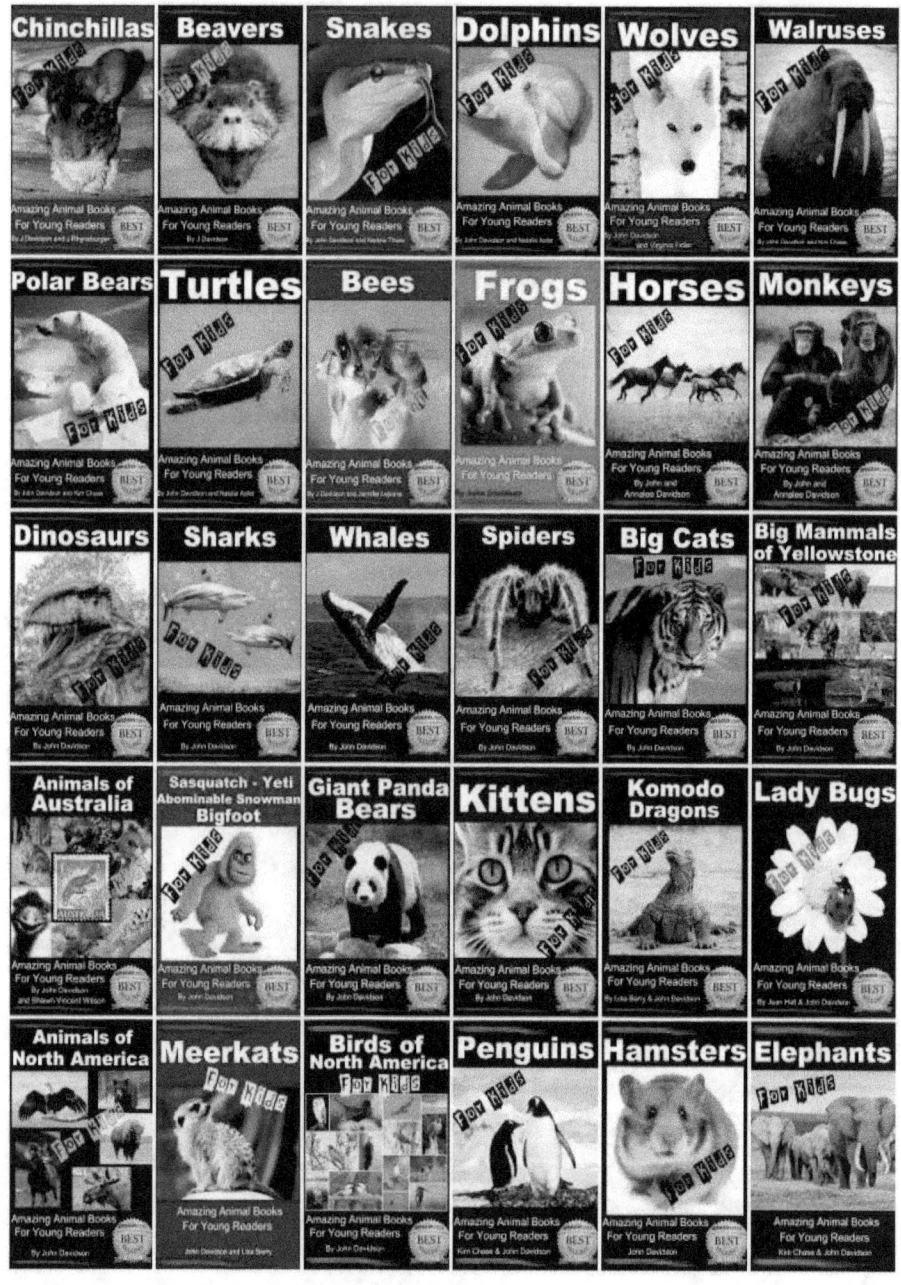

Learn To Draw Series

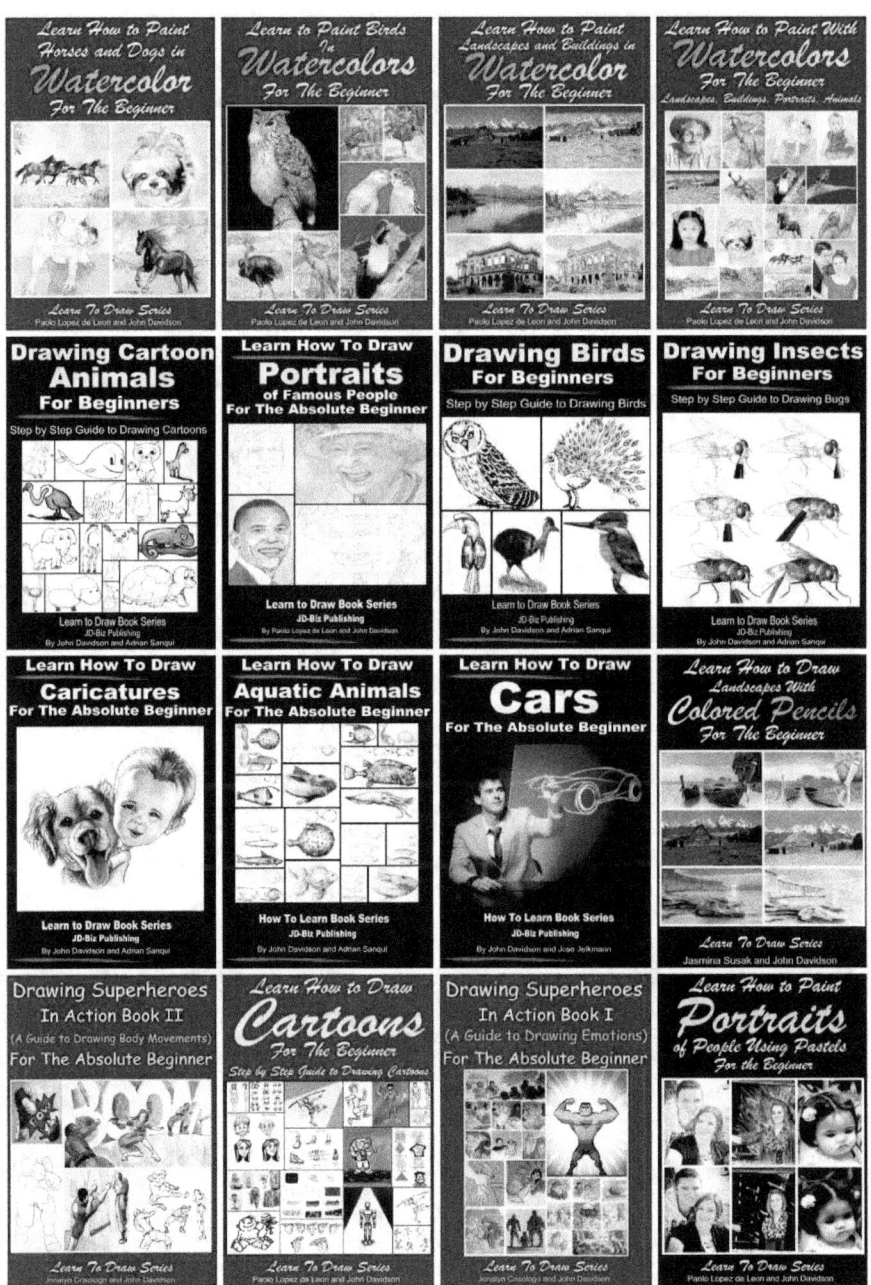

How to Build and Plan Books

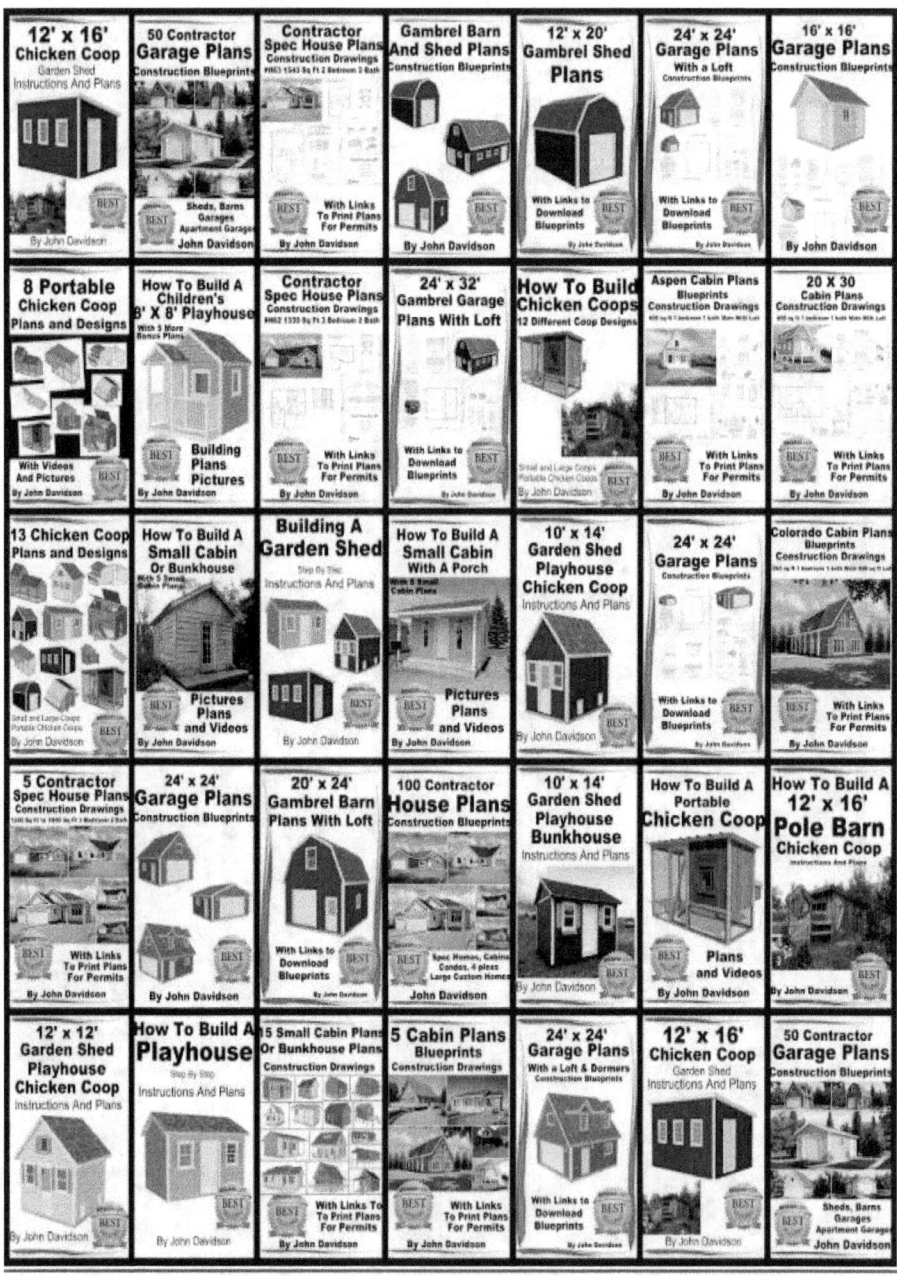

Entrepreneur Book Series

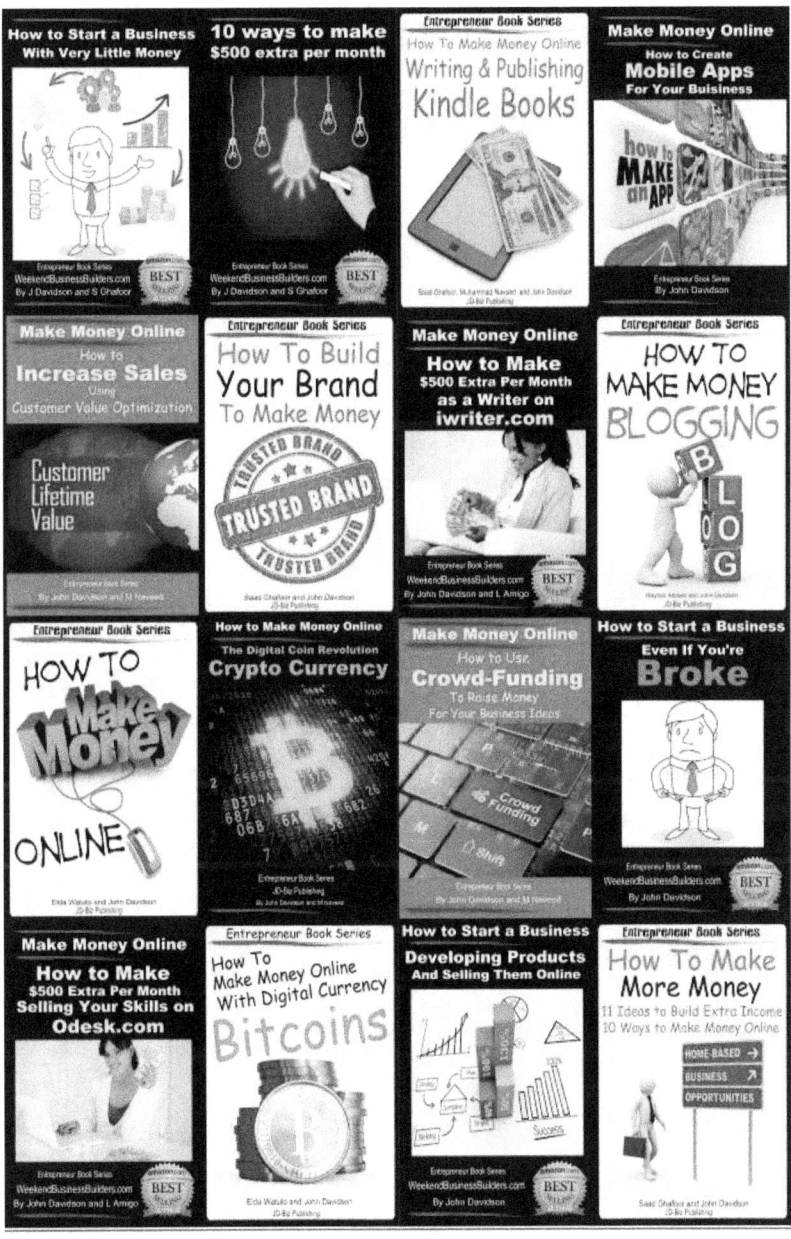

Our books are available at

1. Amazon.com

2. Barnes and Noble

3. Itunes

4. Kobo

5. Smashwords

6. Google Play Books

Publisher

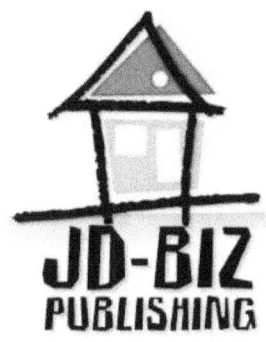

JD-Biz Corp

P O Box 374

Mendon, Utah 84325

http://www.jd-biz.com/

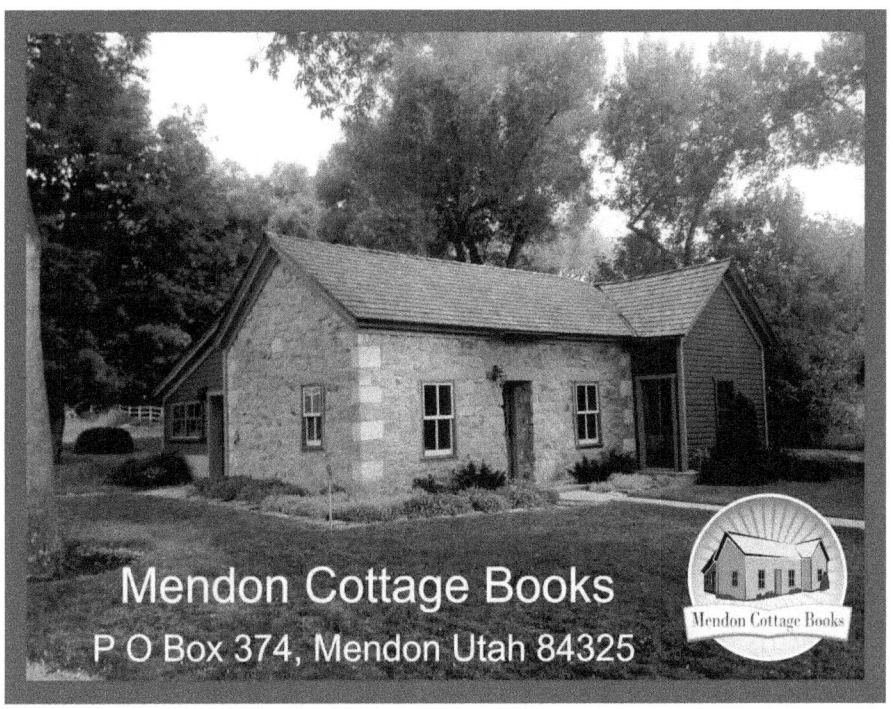

Mendon Cottage Books

P O Box 374, Mendon Utah 84325